Leptin Resistance

Take Control of Your Leptin Hormone with Diet & Supplements to Lose Weight Naturally & Restore Your Health

Christine Weil

Christine Weil

Table of Contents

Introduction

If you are reading this book, chances are that you or a loved one has been diagnosed with Leptin Resistance. Just like with any medical condition, the first and most important steps are to educate yourself on the disorder, learn its effects on the body, and then learn how to manage it.

Congratulations! You have taken the first steps in learning to create a better future and better health. By purchasing **"Leptin Resistance: Take Control of Your Leptin Hormone with Diet & Supplements to Lose Weight Naturally & Restore Your Health,"** you are taking the first step to gaining control of your life and building a healthier, happier you.

Over 50 million people in the United States suffer from this disorder. This means that about one out of every six people are fighting against their own body and their own hormones in their efforts to lose weight and become healthier. They are also fighting a battle with diet and portion size. They are fighting with their body to control hunger cravings and the need to snack.

No matter how you look at it, your body sending signals of hunger all the time is just not fair to you. Your own body forcing you to eat, or telling you that unhealthy portion sizes are necessary for you to be comfortable is completely ridiculous, and only YOU can put a stop to it.

Within the pages of this book, you will develop a full understanding of Leptin Resistance, as well as strategies for controlling and reversing the resistance your body has built.

This guide provides information on how to holistically manage this disorder on a natural level and in combination with medications your doctor may prescribe.

I am here to tell you how to take control of your Leptin levels and your resistance, and to become a healthier, happier you that can stand proud.

Thank you for purchasing this book. I hope you are able to develop a great understanding of Leptin Resistance and how to treat your body in a holistic manner to control the effects of this disorder on your body.

Let's dive in together! You are not alone. Together, we are going to show your body who is boss and send it packing for good!

Christine Weil

What is Leptin and Leptin Resistance?

The human body is full of hormones. Hormones control your feelings, keep you safe, tell you what your body needs to stay healthy, determine your height, weight, physical attributes, and they can also be the reason your weight is out of control.

Society typically views people who are overweight as impulse eaters. They also are under the misconception that every person who is overweight or obese has made poor decisions that were under their control. This is not always the case! Yes, there are some people who are overweight because of their own choices, just like there are some people who are unbelievably thin for the same reason.

Because of certain hormones, not everyone who carries around excess weight has made the decision to consume the necessary amount of food to get to this point. In some, only the choice of the type of food can be controlled. No matter what you are eating, if your body is constantly demanding food, you are going to put on excess weight. What is really going on inside your body to cause this weight gain? Let's look at one of the main culprit behind excessive weight loss, the hormone Leptin.

What is Leptin?

Leptin is a hormone in the body that helps to curb your appetite. It is also responsible for controlling metabolism.

The weight loss industry wants you to believe that it is the obesity hormone. The truth is actually quite opposite. Leptin is a starvation hormone, a protein that is created in fat cells. This protein circulates through your bloodstream and makes its way to your brain. It tells the brain that your body has built up enough energy storage in your fat cells to function on a normal level. It is believed that the actual level of energy your body sees as normal is genetically determined.

When you are on a diet or your body has slowly built a resistance to leptin, you do not take in as much food. You are no longer taking in the levels of 'energy' your brain is used to receiving. It goes into starvation mode instantly. Your brain is not receiving the amount of leptin it expects, which is referred to as your personal threshold. Your brain sets out to bring your level back up to a point it is used to.

Your brain sends out a signal which first targets the vagus nerve, or the energy storage nerve. This nerve runs between your brain and your abdomen. Once this nerve is activated, you begin to feel hungry. The longer your brain is ignored, the hungrier you get. Your brain's intention is for you to take on more food and store more fat, which creates more leptin to bring levels back up to your personal threshold.

So if your body is supposed to shut off hunger when you are full, why do you keep gaining weight?

Just like with any hormone, your body may not produce enough to trigger the "full" response. It can also build up a resistance to this hormone, which means that your brain is not able to process the hormone levels to trigger the "I'm full response."

There are many disorders that can be treated using over the counter supplements. For instance, insomnia can be treated with over the counter melatonin, and other disorders function in the same way.

Unfortunately, while treating someone who is Leptin Resistant with supplements might make sense to some, supplements are not effective, as the body cannot use any of the leptin you eat. Supplementing with Leptin via intramuscular injection does not work unless the person being treated is deficient.

Consuming Foods Containing Leptin

With most medical conditions, you can monitor the level of the needed chemical that can be found in your foods. Unfortunately, consuming foods that contain Leptin will not assist you in the matter of Resistance.

The digestive tract is not able to absorb any form of Leptin to increase your personal levels. Searching for foods that contain it and adding them to your diet will not provide any benefit. In order to be effective, your body must create its own and respond to it. You do not want high levels in your body; this can increase the resistance and ultimately do more damage to the receptors that trigger you feeling full.

The goal is to teach your body to respond to Leptin, and to do so at a lower level.

What is Leptin Resistance?

Leptin is the hormone that controls metabolism and also curbs your appetite. When your brain reads that there is not enough of this chemical in your body to keep it satisfied, it must get your attention. To do so, your body carries out a series of triggers that create hunger.

Unfortunately, your body cannot pull the Leptin it needs from food, so searching for a food that contains it serves no purpose. Basically, what you eat becomes fat, and the fat produces the chemical, which is then released into your blood stream. Once a certain amount is built up in your blood stream, your brain should turn off the hunger response. When someone is resistant to leptin, their brain does not turn off the hunger response even when they are full.

When you have an abnormal increase in the level of leptin in your blood stream over a long period of time, your body learns to ignore it, which results in Leptin insensitivity, in the same manner the levels of insulin can be ignored in diabetics. Not everyone creates their own Resistance. Genetics can also cause your body to be less responsive to the levels in your blood, in turn decreasing your metabolism, increasing your food cravings, and causing you to gain weight.

The key is to work with your body to increase the sensitivity to the hormone Leptin so that you are able to maintain a higher metabolic rate and control your appetite, even if the level of Leptin in your blood were to drop.
Body fat causes the level of Leptin in your body to increase. Carrying around more weight over a long period of time allows your body to build up a higher threshold for the hormone.

Seems like a catch-22 right? How can you get your leptin hormone levels under control when your brain is telling your body that even though you are unhealthy, the weight you are is the weight you should be?

While there are no foods that your body can draw leptin from, there are foods that you can eat to make your body more sensitive to its own levels.

Leptin Resistance and Diabetes

Studies have shown that people who have Leptin Resistance are at increased risk for developing type II diabetes. It is thought that the correlation is due to increased food consumption. The more food you eat, the more insulin your body has to create to keep your blood sugar at a healthy level.

Repeatedly consuming large amounts of food increases your blood sugar. In doing this, your body learns to accept higher and higher blood sugars, because your pancreas cannot keep up with the amount of insulin that your body needs. Once your body becomes "okay" with a higher blood sugar on a regular basis, it triggers your pancreas to create less insulin to compensate, leaving your blood sugar uncontrolled, and leaving your body in a very unhealthy state.

It is important to note that not everyone who is diabetic will develop Leptin Resistance, and not everyone who is Leptin Resistant will develop diabetes.

Those who have Leptin Resistance develop abnormal amounts of fat mass. This is caused by over-eating dietary toxins like wheat, sugar, frying oils, and other unhealthy foods. As the amount of fat in the body increases, the brain becomes immune to the Leptin in releases. It no longer realizes that the body has taken in enough fat to sustain energy, so more and more fat is allowed through.

If extremely high Leptin levels are constantly soaring through the blood, the brain learns to completely ignore the hormone because it is always there. Over time, Leptin Resistance allows large amounts of free fatty acids to deposit outside of the designated deposit locations into other tissues nearby, where fat cells are not supposed to be. This fat then begins to damage the surrounding tissue.

The longer Leptin Resistance is present, the more fat cells grow and the larger they become. When cells become larger than their cell walls are meant to sustain, they develop an instability and rupture. When the cell ruptures, their contents deposit in the tissue, and the body tries its best to clean them up. Unfortunately, it is not able to clean up all of the dead and dying fat cells.

What is left from the cells sets a condition called lipotoxicity and inflammation. Over time, this toxicity begins affecting the pancreas which results in insulin resistance, or type II diabetes.

Who is Susceptible to Leptin Resistance?

Those who are susceptible to Leptin Resistance are unfortunately some of the same people who are susceptible to developing diabetes.

If you have eaten a diet that is full of processed foods, sugar, and eating unhealthy portions.

Other risk factors include:

Family history of Leptin Resistance
Family history of obesity
Personal history of obesity
A sedentary lifestyle
Eating disorders
Lack of regular exercise
Long term high stress levels

Symptoms of Leptin Resistance

- High Body Mass Index
- Increased stress
- Irritably
- Mood swings
- Nocturnal cravings of carbohydrates
- A large appetite
- Over-eating regularly
- High triglycerides
- High cholesterol
- High blood sugar
- Thyroid problems
- Fatty liver
- Fatigue
- Insomnia
- Allergies
- Food sensitivities
- Acne
- Ovarian cysts
- Endometriosis

Diagnostic Process of Leptin Resistance

There are a lot of tests your doctor can do to determine whether or not you are Leptin Resistant. First, s/he will perform a physical examination, and ask you a lot of questions about your eating habits, the way you feel, and they will try to determine whether or not you have the symptoms of this disorder, or if your symptoms fit a different problem.

After your doctor has taken your history and completed a physical examination s/he will then order blood tests. Many of these tests can be used to diagnose other medical problems that have similar symptoms.

The Lab Tests Your Doctor Will Perform

Fasting blood sugar A1C – This test will allow the doctor to determine your average blood sugars over the previous three months. This will show them whether you typically have a higher blood sugar than a healthy person does. The typical AC1 level of a person with Leptin Resistance ranges above 5.6.

Homosysteine and C-Reactive Protein – These blood tests check for cardiovascular disease and whether you are at risk for heart disease. CRP also measures levels of inflammation inside your body. Both heart disease risk and inflammation are indicators of leptin resistance.

Urine Test – Markers in your urine will help your doctor determine whether the proteins in your urine are indicative of leptin resistance.

LDL – LDL is bad cholesterol. Those who have, or are at risk for Leptin Resistance typically have higher cholesterol.

TSH – TSH is sort of a catch-all test. It was once thought that this test could rule out thyroid function disorders. Essentially, those who are Leptin Resistant have thyroid problems attached. However, this test does not tell a physician the level of thyroid hormones being released, only what is in the blood. It does not reveal how healthy your thyroid is.

Ultrasound – An ultrasound test is done on three different areas. The liver typically does not contain any fat. In the body of a healthy person, it is muscle, with a few glands and a vascular system. For a person with Leptin Resistance, an ultrasound will show fat build-up around the liver. The ultrasound technician will also check body fat concentration. Those who suffer from Leptin Resistance develop larger fat cells and fat pockets outside of designated deposit locations.

Women who have Leptin Resistance are more prone to ovarian cysts and cysts inside the uterine wall; this is another location that the ultrasound technician will check.

If your doctor determines that you do have Leptin Resistance, or that you are beginning to develop the disorder, they may prescribe medications to help treat the condition. There are typically two medications that are prescribed for treatment of Leptin Resistance. These two medications are commonly used to treat diabetes and the excessive weight that comes along with it.
Byetta – A diabetic medication that is injectable. It does have certain restrictions and should not be used in combination with certain drugs or disorders. It is commonly prescribed as an "off label" medication to treat Leptin Resistance.

Symlin – An injectable medication used to treat diabetes. However, it can be used off label to help reduce weight and fat in those who have Leptin Resistance.

Even though these medications are authorized for treatment of diabetes, they can be prescribed "off label" to treat Leptin Resistance. The two medications are both used to treat diabetes, but they are also showing a lot of promise in treating the non-diabetic population in stimulating weight loss in those who are overweight.

It is important to note that these drugs do not actually contain leptin, but are used as weight loss agents which remove excess fat from the body. The purpose of removing the excess fat is to deprive the brain of enough leptin to catch it's attention, and reprogram it to the markers found in the hormone.

There are currently no medications that are used specifically for Leptin Resistance. However, there are some changes that can be made in lifestyle and diet that can assist in treating Leptin Resistance. There are also some natural supplements that can be used.

Treating Leptin Resistance Naturally

While there are some medications to treat Leptin Resistance, often the most effective way to treat a problem with the body is naturally. Even if you are on medications prescribed by your doctor, taking a natural approach alongside treatment can improve the outcome of your situation and allow you to gain faster control of your situation.

Exercise

While the prescription medications that are given for Leptin Resistance are aimed at treating the associated weight gain, they are not able to reverse it, or to treat the underlying issue. Since Leptin Supplements do not help, due to your digestive system being unable to extract this chemical from your daily intake, exercise becomes one of the most effective treatments for Leptin Resistance.

Exercise helps reduce Leptin Resistance by increasing serotonin levels in the brain and by burning the excess fat that your brain is ignoring. Burning this fat allows your leptin levels to come down. This may make you feel hungry more often, and may make you want to eat more. However, following a diet plan can help you lose weight, and take control of your leptin levels as well.

The key to treating leptin is to slowly allow your brain less and less Leptin, and bring it back in tune to the chemical in general. For a long time, your brain has been ignoring the levels of Leptin coursing through your blood stream. Once you begin depriving it of Leptin, it will take notice that there has been a major change, and over time, it will adjust to lower and lower levels of this hormone.

If you are not able to withstand high impact exercise, such as cardio, you can start with any exercise. Walking is a great starter exercise. Joining water aerobics will allow you to burn fat without damaging your joints or causing yourself any undue pain.

Keeping up on your exercise, and slowly increasing the duration and frequency, will allow you to burn the excess fat that is releasing Leptin into your body.

In order to curb your cravings while you are depriving your brain of high levels of Leptin, you need to have a great diet plan in order, and you need to follow it completely.

Leptin Resistance Diet

There are many foods that you should eat while on a Leptin Resistant diet. There are also foods that you should eat in moderation or not at all while on this diet. Essentially, you are aiming for a low fat, low cholesterol, low carbohydrate, and high protein diet.

There is a cheat sheet at the end of this book that contains three tables.

The first table is foods you should focus on. The second table is foods you should avoid for the first three weeks of your diet, and the third table contains foods you should avoid completely to reduce your Leptin Levels.

Your diet should contain at least 1,200 calories per day. No matter how desperate you are to lose weight and take back control of your life, you should never consume less than 1,200 calories per day.

You should try to focus mostly on plant-based foods throughout the day. Snacking on vegetables is a great way to curb cravings and to manage your caloric intake, especially if you are used to taking in larger amounts of food than the recommended serving size.

Tips for Cooking

Vegetables

Vegetables have the most nutritional value when they are raw. Once they are cooked, they tend to lose a lot of the benefits they provide to your body. Vegetables should be steamed, and only cooked enough to bring out their flavor. The best way to cook them is through steaming and not through boiling, sautéing, or microwaving. These methods will over-cook the vegetable and will reduce the nutritional value.

Cooked vegetables should not be mushy. Vegetables that still retain resistance when you bite into them take longer to digest, which in turn keeps you full longer.

Meats

Red meats should be cooked to medium well and should never be well done. This is because beyond medium well, the meat begins to lose nutrients, and the protein levels begin to drop. Chicken and pork should always be well done because they contain more bacteria which can be dangerous to your health if they are not cooked through.

Using a counter top grill can be very beneficial, an outdoor grill is not. Charred foods, while delicious, pose serious health risks and increase your risk of developing cancer. While you are trying to solve one problem, there is no need to create another.

Length of Diet

This diet should *not* be followed long term. It is a short-term diet only that should be followed for a maximum of six weeks at a time. The diet can be done more than once, but you should always have a 2 week rest period between diet phases. By following a strict diet and exercise regimen, you will be able to reset the leptin receptors in your brain to pay more attention to the levels in your blood.

Healing From the Inside Out

Healing your body from Leptin Resistance does not just include physically healing. It includes emotional healing as well. It involves finding inner peace and finding a new you. This can be a very emotional time in your life, and making sure that you have the right support system is very important.

There are many things that you can do to ensure that you are healing yourself as a whole. Meditation, acupuncture, massage, reflex therapy, and sometimes counseling may be necessary to help you along your journey to finding a new you.

Meditation

Stress can increase the urge to eat, increase the amount of leptin in your blood, and increase your blood pressure. It is very important that you take time to rid your body of stress and feel better about yourself.

Meditation is great for your health, great for your mind, and great for your spirit. It allows you time to reflect on your emotions and manage them in a healthy way. You can learn to manage the emotions and the way your body feels from day to day.

One of the most important things you can do on your journey to reversing leptin resistance is to pay attention to your body. You are making a dramatic change in your life which can become an emotional roller coaster. It is important for you to manage your emotions as they come, and to not ignore them.

Not only are you healing yourself physically, but you are healing yourself emotionally as well. You are creating a new life, and you are shedding a lot of weight. Coming to terms with the changes occurring in your body can be made a lot easier by creating an inner peace.

Acupuncture

Over the last several years, there have been reports of people overcoming Leptin Resistance with a combination of diet, exercise, meditation, and acupuncture. If you are a believer in natural and alternative medicine, you may find a great deal of benefit in a routine acupuncture visit.

Acupuncture releases negative energy from your body, releases pain, and relieves inflammation. It can be very relaxing. Since pain and inflammation are major factors in Leptin Resistance, you may notice a substantial change in your ability to get up and move around, which makes exercise easier and less painful.

Massage

Along your journey to find a healthier, smaller you, massage may be extremely beneficial. Exercise can be difficult and very painful if you are heavier and are overcoming years of weight gain.

Massage not only helps relieve pain, but it also makes you feel better about yourself and your ability to overcome your circumstances. Make sure that your massage therapist has worked with people who have had Leptin Resistance or diabetes.

Reflexology

When most people think of reflexology, they think of treatment for the immune system, or even getting reflexology to assist in comfort in the early stages of labor. However, reflexology has much more to offer, especially now that you are going through a total body change.

Since excess fatty tissue in the body can cause your immune system to become weak, reflexology is able to help with inflammation and with building your immune system back up while you work on getting rid of the excess weight. You do not have to wait until your transformation is complete to start reflexology. You can begin both your journey and reflexology at the same time.

Supplements for Reversing Leptin Resistance

While there are no supplements containing leptin that benefit the human body, there are some that make it easier to create leptin and process it. These are supplements like omega-3s, dietary fiber, zinc, and melatonin.

Omega-3s – these fatty acids help adjust leptin sensitivity. They help the brain recognize chemicals in the brain at lower levels. You should not ingest too much omega-3 fatty acids. The limit should be no more than 3 grams per day.

Dietary Fiber – Fiber helps break down fat and flush out impurities. It also helps reduce cholesterol and burns fat at a faster rate. While most foods are not a great source of dietary fiber, you can use fiber supplements to increase your daily intake. These supplements can be in the form of capsules, pills, and drink mixes.

Zinc – Zinc is a mineral that helps the brain recognize leptin. It can be taken in the form of a standalone vitamin, or in the form of a multi-vitamin.

Melatonin – Melatonin is a natural sleep aid. It is a chemical found naturally in the brain that helps you fall asleep. Taking a melatonin supplement can increase your quality of sleep. Getting enough sleep, and enough quality sleep can greatly impact your ability to process certain chemicals in your brain.

Water – While water isn't a supplement, in this case, it can be. A dehydrated body does not burn fat at the same rate that a hydrated body does. Water helps flush away excess chemicals, hormones, and build up from the body. Staying hydrated can dramatically increase your ability regulate your leptin levels.

Recipes for a Leptin-Resistant Diet

Choosing your food wisely is the best way to control your Leptin levels and retrain your brain to respond to your own chemistry. Here are a few recipes to get you started.

Raspberry Vanilla Oatmeal

Ingredients

- 3/4 cup uncooked oats
- 1/2 cup almond milk or organic 2% milk
- 1/4 - 1/2 scoop protein powder
- 1 Tbsp. date paste (2 or 3 dates blended in water)
- frozen or fresh raspberries to taste
- 1/2 tsp vanilla extract or powder
- dash of Himalayan salt
- almonds, walnuts, or other nut of choice to garnish
- purified water, to cover mixture

Instructions

1. Mix ingredients, except nuts, and refrigerate overnight.

2. Serve cold or warm.

3. Top with more raspberries and nuts of your choice.

Avocado Mango Salad with Chili Lime Vinaigrette

Ingredients

- 1/2 jalapeño chili, seeded and minced
- Juice of 2 limes
- 1/4 cup olive oil
- 1/2 tsp. coarse sea salt
- Freshly ground pepper, to taste
- 1 mango
- 1 avocado
- 6 cups organic mixed salad greens

Instructions

1. To make the vinaigrette: combine the jalapeño and lime juice in a small bowl.

2. Whisk in the olive oil.

3. Season with salt and pepper.

4. Set aside until ready to serve.

5. Cube flesh of avocado and mango.

6. Toss salad greens, avocado, mango, and vinaigrette.

Makes 4 servings.

Seared Salmon with Roasted Asparagus

Ingredients

- 4 servings wild Alaskan salmon fillet

(about 1 1/4 pounds total)

- 1 Tbsp. chopped fresh rosemary or 1 teaspoon dried
- 1 teaspoon salt
- 1 - 1 1/2 pounds fresh organic asparagus
- 1 1/2 Tbsp. extra-virgin olive oil
- 1 small organic onion, diced
- 2 tablespoons pine nuts
- 1 cup filtered water
- 1/2 cup brown rice

Instructions

1. Preheat oven to 425 degrees.

2. Season salmon with half the rosemary and 1/2 teaspoon salt for 20 minutes, up to 1 hour before cooking.

3. Start preparing brown rice. Add 1 cup filtered water to pot and bring to a boil. Add 1/2 cup brown rice to water, set to low, and cover. Rice will be done in 35-40 minutes.

4. Snap the bottom of the asparagus ends. Season asparagus with 1/2 teaspoon salt and some olive oil, toss to combine. Bake the asparagus for about 8-10 minutes at 425 degrees.

5. Heat 1 tablespoon oil in a large wide saucepan over medium heat. Add diced onion, and cook, stirring occasionally, until translucent, 3 to 4 minutes. Add pine nuts and the remaining rosemary. Cook, stirring, until the pine nuts are fragrant, and are beginning to brown, 3 to 5 minutes.

6. Meanwhile, heat the remaining oil in a large nonstick skillet over medium-high heat. Add salmon, skinned-side up, and cook until golden brown, 3 to 5 minutes. Turn the salmon over, remove the pan from the heat and let stand until just cooked through, 3 to 5 minutes more.

7. Serve with a scoop of brown rice on bottom, topped with salmon. Spoon pine nuts and any liquid remaining in the pan over the salmon.

Healthy Yogurt Parfait

Ingredients

- 1 cup Organic Plain Yogurt (antibiotics and hormone-free)
- ¼ cup Organic Raw Granola (no sweetener)
- ¼ cup Organic Goji Berries (dried)
- Organic Honey, optional, if more sweetness is desired

Instructions

Add in some of the granola, goji berries, and optional honey to your yogurt, and mix well. Put in serving dish, and top with the rest of your granola and goji berries.

Serves 2.

Cucumber Mint Cooler

Ingredients

- 1 scoop Daily Protein Unflavored
- 1 cup chopped, seeded, and peeled cucumber
- 1/4 cup chopped fresh mint
- 1 cup water
- 1 teaspoon honey
- Ice cubes

Instructions

Combine the ingredients in a blender; process until smooth.

Leptin Resistant Diet Cheat Sheet

This cheat sheet will guide you through the diet you will need to follow to reverse your Leptin Resistance.

Foods You Should Focus On (Table 1)

Fats	
Nuts and Nut Butters	Nuts and nut butters should be raw, unroasted an unsalted. Peanuts, since they are legumes and not true nuts, should be avoided.
A serving size of almonds, or 23 nuts.	
A serving size of brazil nuts, or 8 nuts.	
A serving size of cashews, or 23 nuts	
A serving size of hazelnuts, or 8 nuts.	
A serving size of macadamia nuts, or 12 nuts.	
A serving size of pecans, or 10 nuts.	
A serving size of pine nuts, or one tablespoon.	
A serving size of pistachios, or 49 nuts.	
A serving size of walnuts, or 18 halves.	
Fruits	The best fruits to eat are avocado and Olives. These fruits contain many health benefits and also provide healthy fats.
Olives	A serving size of olives is between 3 and 5 olives, depending on their size.

Avocado	A serving size of avocado is about 1/5th of an avocado. If you are eating guacamole, you should eat no more than ¼ cup of avocado.
Oils	Oils should be low in saturated fat and should not be commercially processed.
Olive Oil	Foods that are cooked with olive oil should only be cooked with 1 tbsp of oil.
Almond Oil	Foods that are cooked in almond oil should only be cooked with 1 tbsp of oil.
Avocado Oil	Foods that are cooked in avocado should only be cooked with 1 tbsp of oil.

Proteins

Fish (highest in omega-3 Fatty acids)	Omega-3s are considered poly-unsaturated fats. They are easier for the body to break down and assist in flushing unhealthy fat from the body. They do not clog arteries and they provide great cardiovascular and muscle benefits.
Halibut	One serving of halibut is 4 ounces when it is raw, or a piece that is about the size of a deck of cards. It contains approximately 125 calories, 36 mg of cholesterol, contains 23.5 grams of protein, contains 53.1 grams of calcium, and 508.5 mg of potassium.
Herring	One serving size of herring is 229 calories, 87 mg of cholesterol, 26 grams of protein, 83.5 mg of calcium, and 473.5 mg of potassium.
Mackerel	Canned Mackerel: A serving size is one cube size from the can. It contains 25 calories, 13

	mg of cholesterol, no carbs, no dietary fiber, no sugars, 3.7 g of protein, 38 mg of calcium and 31 mg of potassium. Fresh Mackerel: The serving size is 4 ounces when raw. One serving size contains 119 calories, 60 mg of cholesterol, 179 mg of sodium, no carbs, no dietary fiber, 23 g of protein, 35 mg of calcium, and 491.6 mg of potassium.
Orange Roughy	A serving size of orange roughy is approximately 4 ounces. It is about the size of a deck of cards when raw. It contains 86 calories, 68 mg of cholesterol, 81 mg of sodium, 18.5 g of protein, 10.2 mg of calcium, and 188.7 mg of potassium.
Sardines	Canned sardines packed in their own oil should be eaten in moderation. One sardine contains 25 calories, 17 mg of cholesterol, 61 mg of sodium, 3 g of protein, 45 mg of calcium, and 47 mg of potassium.
Tuna	Canned Tuna (light in water): 1 serving size is 1 cup of solid tuna or chunks. It contains 179 calories, 46 mg of cholesterol, 521 mg of sodium, 39 g of protein, 16.9 mg of calcium, and 365 mg of potassium. Fresh: A serving size of fresh tuna is approximately 6 ounces before it is cooked. It contains 180 calories, 75 mg of cholesterol, 65 mg of sodium, 40 mg of protein and 20 mh of calcium.
Fish and Seafood	

Bass	Sea Bass: One serving size of sea bass is approximately 4 ounces. The piece of fish should be about the size of a deck of cards. A serving this size has around 110 calories 46 mg of cholesterol, 77 mg of cholesterol, 11 mg calcium, and 289.3 mg.
Catfish	One serving of catfish is about 4 ounces, or the size of a deck of cards. It contains 107 calories, 66 mg of cholesterol, 49 mg of sodium, 18 grams of protein, 15.8 mg of calcium and 405 mg of potassium.
Cod	One serving of Cod is approximately 4 ounces. It has 93 calories, 49 mg of cholesterol, 61 mg of sodium, 20 g of protein, 18 mg of calcium, and 466 mg of potassium.
Crab	Jumbo Lump, Canned: Serving size 2 ounces. Contains 40 calories, 45 mg of cholesterol, 18 mg of sodium, 10 g of protein. Dungeness Crab: Steamed or boiled: Serving size 3 ounces. Contains 94 calories, 65 mg cholesterol, 321 mg sodium, 0.8 carbs, 50.2 mg of calcium, 345 mg potassium. Alaskan King Crab: Serving size 3 ounces. Contains 82 calories, 45 mg cholesterol, 911 mg of sodium, 16 grams protein, 50 mg calcium, 222 mg potassium.
Flounder	A serving size of flounder is approximately 4 ounces. It contains 103 calories, 54 mg of cholesterol, 92 mg sodium, no carbs, no dietary fiber, no sugars, 21.3 mg protein, 20 mg calcium, 407 mg of potassium.

Grouper	A serving size of grouper is approximately 4 ounces before it is cooked. It contains 104 calories, 42 mg of cholesterol, 60 mg of sodium, 20 mg of protein, 30 mg of calcium and 545 mg of potassium.
Haddock	A serving size of haddock is approximately 4 ounces. It contains 98 calories, 64 mg cholesterol, 77 mg sodium, 20 grams protein, 37 mg calcium and 351 mg potassium.
Halibut	One serving of halibut is 4 ounces when it is raw, or a piece that is about the size of a deck of cards. It contains approximately 125 calories, 36 mg of cholesterol, contains 23.5 grams of protein, contains 53.1 grams of protein, and 508.5 mg of potassium.
Herring	One serving is about 4 ounces when raw. It is a piece about the size of a deck of cards. One serving size of herring is 229 calories, 87 mg of cholesterol, 26 grams of protein, 83.5 mg of calcium, and 473.5 mg of potassium.
Lobster	A serving of lobster is about 3 ounces. It contains 77 calories, 81 mg of cholesterol, 252 mg of sodium, 0.4 carbs, 16 grams protein, 40 mg calcium, 233 mg of potassium.
Mackerel	Canned Mackerel: A serving size is one cube size from the can. It contains 25 calories, 13 mg of cholesterol, 3.7 g of protein, 38 mg of calcium and 31 mg of potassium. Fresh Mackerel: The serving size is 4 ounces when raw. One serving size contains 119 calories, 60 mg of cholesterol, 179 mg of

	sodium, 23 g of protein, 35 mg of calcium, and 491.6 mg of potassium.
Mahimahi	One serving size of mahimahi is approximately 4 ounces. It contains 90 calories, 40 mg of cholesterol, 95 mg of sodium, 21 g protein,
Orange Roughy	A serving size of orange roughy is approximately 4 ounces. It is about the size of a deck of cards when raw. It contains 86 calories, 68 mg of cholesterol, 81 mg of sodium, 18.5 g of protein, 10.2 mg of calcium, and 188.7 mg of potassium.
Oysters (canned or fresh)	A serving of oysters is approximately 1.8 ounces. It contains 41 calories, 25 mg of cholesterol, 53 mg of cholesterol, 2.5 g of carbs, 4.7 grams of protein, 4 mg of calcium, and 84 mg of potassium. Eastern Oyster, raw: A serving size of raw oysters is approximately ½ ounce. One serving contains 8 calories, 4 mg of cholesterol, 25 mg of sodium, .8 total carbs, .7 g of protein, 6.2 mg of calcium, and 17.4 mg of potassium. Canned boiled oysters: Serving size, 1/3 cup. Each serving contains 70 calories, 35 mg cholesterol, 150 mg of sodium, 4 grams of carbohydrates, and 7 grams of protein.
Perch	A serving size of baked perch is a 1.6 ounces. Each fillet contains 55 calories, 53 mg of cholesterol, 11 g of protein, 45 mg of calcium, 158 mg of potassium.
Pollock	A serving size of Pollock is approximately 4 ounces. It contains 104 calories, 80 mg of cholesterol, 97 mg of sodium, no carbs, no

	dietary fiber, no sugar, 22 g of protein, 67 mg of calcium, and 402 mg of potassium.
Rainbow Trout	A serving size of baked rainbow trout is about 2.5 ounces. It contains 12o calories, 48 mg of cholesterol, 30 mg of sodium, 17 grams of protein, 61 mg of calcium, 313 mg of potassium.
Salmon (canned or fresh)	One serving of Atlantic salmon is approximately 4 ounces. It contains 207 calories, 67 mg of cholesterol, 67 mg of sodium, 22 g of protein, 14 grams of calcium, 409 mg of potassium. Red Salmon: A serving size of red salmon is approximately 1 ounce. Each serving contains 47 calories, 12 mg of cholesterol, 102 mg of sodium, 6 grams of protein, 62 mg of calcium, 80 grams of potassium.
Sardines (canned in water, sardine oil, mustard or olive oil)	Canned sardines packed in their own oil should be eaten in moderation. One sardine contains 25 calories, 17 mg of cholesterol, 61 mg of sodium, 3 g of protein, 45 mg of calcium, and 47 mg of potassium.
Scallops	A serving of scallops is approximately 3 ounces. Each serving contains 75 calories, 28 mg of cholesterol, 2 g of carbs, 14 g of protein, 10 mg calcium, and 270 mg of potassium.
Shrimp (canned or fresh)	A serving size of steamed shrimp is approximately 3 ounces. It contains about 84 calories, 166 mg of cholesterol, 190 mg of

	sodium, 17 g of protein, 33 mg of calcium, 154 mg of potassium.
Snapper	A serving of baked snapper is approximately 4 ounces. It contains 145 calories, 53 mg of cholesterol, 64 mg of sodium, 29 g protein, 45 mg of calcium, and 589 mg of potassium.
Sole	A serving size of sole is approximately 4 ounces. It contains 103 calories, 54 mg of cholesterol, 92 mg sodium, 21.3 mg protein, 20 mg calcium, 407 mg of potassium.
Tilapia	A serving of tilapia is approximately 4 ounces. It contains 145 calories, 3 g of fat, 64 mg of cholesterol, 63 mg of sodium, 29 mg of protein, 15 mg of calcium, 428 mg of potassium.
Tuna (canned or fresh)	Canned Tuna (light in water): 1 serving size is 1 cup of solid tuna or chunks. It contains 179 calories, 46 mg of cholesterol, 521 mg of sodium, 39 g of protein, 16.9 mg of calcium, and 365 mg of potassium. Fresh: A serving size of fresh tuna is approximately 6 ounces before it is cooked. It contains 180 calories, 75 mg of cholesterol, 65 mg of sodium, 40 mg of protein and 20 mg of calcium.
Turbot	Serving size, approximately 4 ounces. Contains 204 calories per serving, 98 mg cholesterol, 306 mg sodium, and 33 grams of protein.
Eggs	Eggs should only be eaten from algae or flax seed fed chicken. It is important to get Omega-3 enriched eggs. It is not always easy to tell how chickens are raised by looking at the packaging. However, there are ways to

tell exactly what you are buying when you are looking for eggs. Follow this simple key and try to buy eggs from organically fed chickens.

helpful key

| caged up in tight quarters | no access to sunlight | access to sunlight | clipped beaks & wings | eats organic | eats bugs & grass |

Poultry (preferably free-range or organic)	**All nutritional information here is represented in the raw state. Please note that any seasonings you add will increase all numerical factors.**
Chicken breast, no skin	The serving size of a piece of chicken breast is approximately 4 ounces, or the size of a deck of cards. It contains 124 calories in its raw state. It also contains 66 mg of cholesterol, 73 mg of sodium, no carbs, no dietary fiber, no sugars, 26 mg of protein, 12.4 mg of calcium, and 288 mg of potassium.
Ground Chicken	A serving of ground chicken breast is approximately 4 ounces. It contains 180 calories. It also contains 90 mg of sodium, no carbs, no dietary fiber, no sugars, 19 grams of protein.
Ground Turkey	A serving size of fat-free ground turkey is approximately 4 ounces. It contains approximately 94 calories, 53 mg of cholesterol, 42 mg of sodium, no carbs, no dietary fiber, 20.9 mg protein, 8 mg calcium, 249 mg potassium.

Chicken Sausage	A serving of chicken sausage yields about 1.6 ounces. It contains 116 calories, 45 mg of cholesterol, 617 mg of sodium, 3.1 carbs, no dietary fiber, no sugars, 5.8 g of protein, 42 mg of calcium, 37 mg of potassium.
Turkey Sausage	A serving of turkey sausage is 2 links. It contains 134 calories, 34 mg of cholesterol, 322 mg of sodium, 0.8 g carbohydrates, no dietary fiber, no sugars, 4.4 g protein, 9.1 mg calcium, 55.8 mg potassium.
Game	
Cornish game hen	The serving size for Cornish game hen is ½ of a bird. This serving size contains 168 calories, 170 mg of cholesterol, 102 mg of sodium, no carbs, no dietary fiber, no sugars and 29 mg of protein.
Buffalo	Serving size 1 patty. Each patty of buffalo meat contains 252 calories, 79 mg of cholesterol, 75 mg of sodium, no carbs, no dietary fiber, no sugars and 21 grams of protein.
Ostrich	A serving size of ground ostrich is approximately 1 patty. Each patty contains 180 calories, 77 mg of cholesterol, 78 mg of sodium, no carbs, no dietary fiber, no sugars, 22 grams of protein.
Pheasant	A serving of pheasant is one breast. Each serving contains 169 calories, 98 mg of cholesterol, 56 mg of sodium, no carbs, no dietary fiber, no sugars, and 41 g of protein.
Rabbit	A serving of 6 ounces of rabbit contains 114 calories. It also contains 81 mg of cholesterol, 50 mg of sodium, no carbs, no

	dietary fiber, no sugars, and 22 grams of protein.
Venison	A serving of 6 ounces of deer meat contains approximately 157 calories, 80 mg of cholesterol, 75 mg of sodium, no carbs, no dietary fiber, and 22 grams of protein.

Veggie Burgers (<7 carbs each)

Morning Star Farms Veggie Sausage	This brand of veggie patties contains about 110 calories per patty. A single patty is a serving. It contains no cholesterol, 350 mg of sodium, 9 g of carbs, 3 g of dietary fiber, 1 g of sugar, 10 g of protein and 180 mg of potassium.
Garden Touch Vegan Veggie Patties	In this brand of veggie patties, each one contains 80 calories, 270 mg of sodium, 12 g carbs, 4 g dietary fiber, no sugar, 9 g protein, 40 mg calcium, and 70 mg of potassium.

Dairy

Goat Cheese	One serving of goat cheese is 1 ounce. There are two recommended kinds of goat cheese. Semi-soft goat cheese One serving of semi-soft goat cheese is 103 calories, 22 mg of cholesterol, 0.7 total carbs, no dietary fiber, 0.7 g, 6.1 g, 6.1 g protein, 84.5 mg calcium, 44 mg of potassium. Soft Goat Cheese

	Ones serving contains 76 calories, 104 mg sodium, 13 mg cholesterol, 0.3 g sugars, 5.3 g protein, 39.7 mg calcium, 7.4 mg potassium.
No-fat cottage cheese	One serving of no fat cottage cheese is approximately ½ cup. It contains 80 calories, 5 mg of cholesterol, 420 mg of sodium, 5 g total carbs, no dietary fiber, no sugars, 14 grams of protein, and 100 mg calcium.
No-fat cream cheese	One serving of cream cheese is approximately 17 calories, it also contains 1 mg of cholesterol, 98 mg of sodium, 1 g of carbs, no dietary fiber, less than 0.1 g, 2.6 grams of protein, 33.3 mg of calcium, 29.3 mg of potassium.
No-fat ricotta cheese	A serving of fat-free ricotta cheese is about ¼ cup. It contains approximately 50 calories, 65 grams of sodium, 5 grams of carbs, no dietary fiber, 2 grams of sugars, protein 5 mg, and 100 mg of calcium.
Feta Cheese	One serving of feta cheese is about 1 ounce. It contains about 75 calories, 25 mg of cholesterol, 316 mg sodium, no dietary fiber, 1.2 grams of cars, no dietary fiber, 1.2 grams of sugar, 4 grams protein, 139 mg of calcium, and 17 mg of potassium.
Light Swiss Cheese	One ounce of light, creamy Swiss cheese is considered a serving size. Each serving contains 47 calories, 6 mg of cholesterol, 284 mg of sodium, 1.4 grams of carbs, no dietary fibers, 1.4 grams sugars, 2.7 grams of protein, and 108 mg of calcium.
Parmesan Cheese (1 tbsp)	One serving of parmesan cheese is 1 tbsp. It contains 22 calories, 4 mg of cholesterol, 76 mg of sodium, 0.2 g carbs, no dietary fiber,

	<0.1 g sugar, 1.9 grams of protein, 55 mg of calcium, 6 mg of potassium.

Dairy

Plain	The serving size for firm tofu is about 2.8 ounces or about 1/5 of a typical sized pack. It contains 70 calories, no cholesterol, no sodium, only 2 grams of carbs, ½ gram of dietary fiber, no sugar, 7 grams of protein and 100 mg of calcium.
Herb	The serving size for firm tofu is about 2.8 ounces or about 1/5 of a typical sized pack. It contains 70 calories, no cholesterol, no sodium, only 2 grams of carbs, ½ gram of dietary fiber, no sugar, 7 grams of protein and 100 mg of calcium.
Flavored (Italian, Oriental, Thai)	The serving size for firm tofu is about 2.8 ounces or about 1/5 of a typical sized pack. It contains 70 calories, no cholesterol, no sodium, only 2 grams of carbs, ½ gram of dietary fiber, no sugar, 7 grams of protein and 100 mg of calcium.

Protein Powder

Egg protein powder	1 scoop of egg protein powder is a serving size. It contains 130 calories, 15 mg cholesterol, 420 mg of sodium, 5 g carbs, 1 g dietary fiber, 1 g sugars, 24 g protein.
Vegetable protein	The serving size for vegetable protein powder is about 2 rounded tbsp. It contains 80 calories, no cholesterol, 200 mg sodium, no carbs, no sugars, no dietary fiber, and 17 grams of protein.

Whey Protein	The serving size for whey protein powder is about 1 scoop. It contains 110 calories, 35 mg of cholesterol, 55 mg of sodium, 175 mg of potassium, 1 g carbs, no dietary fiber, 1 g sugars, and 23 g protein.

Carbohydrates (All numeric values are given for raw vegetable)

Asparagus	Serving size: 1 cup Each serving contains 27 calories, no cholesterol, 0.2 g of fat, 271 mg of sodium, 5.2 g carbohydrates, 2.8 g dietary fiber, 2.5 g of sugars, and 2.9 g of protein.
Artichoke hearts	Serving size: 1 cup. Each serving contains 58 calories, no cholesterol, 1.9 grams of fat, 280 mg of sodium, 297 grams of potassium, 9 grams of carbs, 4 g of dietary fiber, 0.83 g of sugars, and 2.9 g of protein,
Arugula	Serving size: 1 cup. Each serving contains 5 calories, 0.1 g of fat, no cholesterol, 4 mg of sodium, 74 mg of potassium, 0.73 g of carbs, 0.3 grams of dietary fiber, 0.41 g of sugar, 0.52 g of protein.
Bamboo Shoots	Serving size: 1 cup. Each serving size has 41 calories, 0.45 g of fat, 0 mg of cholesterol, 6 mg of sodium, 805 mg of potassium, 7.85 g carbohydrates, 3 grams dietary fiber, 4 grams sugars, and 3.9 grams of protein.
Bell peppers	Serving size: 1 cup. One serving contains 31 calories, 0.36 g total fat, no cholesterol, 3 mg sodium, 251 mg potassium, 7.18 g carbs, 2.4 g dietary fiber, 5 g sugars, and 1.18 g protein.
Bok Choy	Serving Size: 1 cup shredded. Each serving contains 9 calories, 0.14 g fat, no cholesterol, 46 mg sodium, 176 mg potassium, 1.53 g carbs, 0.7 g dietary fiber, 0.83 g sugars, and 1.05 g protein.

Broccoli	Serving size: 1 cup chopped. Each serving contains 31 calories, 0.34 g fat, 0 cholesterol, 30 mg sodium, 288 mg potassium, 6.04 g total carbs, 2.4 g dietary fiber, 1.5 g sugar, 2.57 g protein.
Brussels Sprouts	Serving size: 1 cup. Each serving contains 38 calories, 0.26g of fat, no cholesterol, 22 mg sodium, 342 mg potassium, 7.88 g carbs, 3.3 g dietary fiber, and 1.98 g protein.
Cabbage	Serving size: 1 cup chopped. Each serving contains 21 calories, 0.11 g total fat, no cholesterol, 16 mg sodium, 219 mg potassium, 4.97 g total carbs, 2 g dietary fiber, 3.29 g sugars, and 1.28 g total protein.
Cauliflower	Serving size, 1 cup. Each cup of cauliflower contains 25 calories, 0.1 g fat, no cholesterol, 30 mg of sodium, 303 mg of potassium, 5.3 total carbohydrates, 2.5 g dietary fiber, 2.4 g sugars, 1.98 g protein.
Celery	Serving size, 1 medium stalk. Each serving contains 6 calories, no fat, no cholesterol, 32 mg of sodium, 104 mg of potassium, 1.19 carbohydrates, no dietary fiber, no sugars, and 0.28 g of protein.
Chard	Serving Size: 1 cup. Each cup of chard contains 7 calories, no cholesterol, 77 mg of sodium, 136 mg of potassium, 1.35 g carbs, 0.5 g dietary fiber, 0.4 g sugars, and 0.65 g protein.
Chives	Serving size: 1 tbsp. Each tablespoon of chopped chives contains 1 calorie, 0.02 grams total fat, no cholesterol, no sodium, 9 mg of potassium, 0.13 g carbs, no dietary fiber, no sugars, and 0.1 g protein.
Cilantro	Serving size: 1 sprig. Each serving size has no calories, 0.1 g total fat, no cholesterol, 1

	mg sodium, 0.04 total carbs, 6 mg of potassium, no sugars, no dietary fiber, and 0.02 grams protein.
Cucumbers	Serving size: 1 cup peeled. One serving contains 16 calories, 0.21 grams fat, no cholesterol, 3 mg sodium, 181 mg potassium, 2.87 g total carbs, 0.8 g total dietary fiber, 1.84 g sugars, and 0.78g protein.
Eggplant	Serving size: 1 cup. Each serving has 20 calories, 0.16 grams fat, no cholesterol, 2 mg sodium, 189 mg potassium, 4.67 g carbs, 2.8 g dietary fiber, 1.93 g sugars, and 0.83 g protein.
Fennel	Serving size 1 fennel bulb. Each serving has 33 calories, no cholesterol, 187 mg sodium, 608 mg potassium, 6.9 g carbs, 3.7 g dietary fiber, 4.28 g sugars, and 1.61 g protein.
Greens (collard, turnip, mustard, chard)	Collards: One serving size: 1 cup: Each serving contains 11 calories, 0.15 g fat, no cholesterol, 7 mg sodium, 2.04 g total carbs, 1.3 g dietary fiber, 0.17 g sugars, and 0.88 g protein. Turnip: One Serving: 1 cup chopped. Each serving contains 18 calories, 0.16 g fat, no cholesterol, 22 mg sodium, 163 mg potassium, 3.82 g carbs, 1.8 g dietary fiber, 0.45 g sugars, and 0.82 g protein. Mustard: One Serving: 1 cup chopped. Each serving contains 15 calories, 0.11 grams fat, no cholesterol, 15 mg sodium, 198 mg potassium, 2.74 g carbs, 1.8 g dietary fiber, 0.9 g sugars, 1.51 g protein.

Hot Peppers	Serving size: 1 pepper. Each pepper contains 18 calories, 0.08 g total fat, 0 mg cholesterol, 3 mg sodium, 153 mg potassium, 4.26 g carbs, 0.7 g dietary fiber, 2.3 g sugars, 0.9 g protein.
Kale	Serving size: 1 cup chopped. Each cup of kale contains 34 calories, 0.47 g fat, 0 mg cholesterol, 29 mg sodium, 299 mg potassium, 6.71 g total carbs, 1.3 g dietary fiber, no sugars, 2.21 g protein.
Kohlrabi	Serving size: 1 cup. Each serving contains 36 calories, 0.14 g fat, no cholesterol, 27 mg sodium, 472 mg potassium, 8.37 g carbs, 4.9 g dietary fiber, 3.51 g sugars, 2.3 g protein.
Lettuce (not iceberg)	Serving Size: 1 cup of shredded or chopped. Each serving contains 8 calories, 0.08 g fat, no cholesterol, 6 mg sodium, 78 mg potassium, 1.63 g carbs, 0.7 g dietary fiber, 0.97 g sugars, 0.5 g protein.
Leeks	Serving size: 1 ounce. Each serving of leeks contains 17 calories, 0.09 g of fat, no cholesterol, 6 mg sodium, 51 mg potassium, 4.01 g total carbs, 0.5 g dietary fiber, 1.11 g sugars, 0.43 g protein,
Mushrooms (Portobello, shitake, oyster, button)	Portobello: Serving size, 1 cap. Calories 20, no fat, no cholesterol 15 mg sodium, 300 mg potassium, 3 g carbs, 1 g dietary fiber, no sugars, and 3 g of protein. Shiitake: Serving size ½ cup. Each serving contains 30 calories, 1 g fat, no cholesterol, 620 mg sodium, no potassium, 4 g carbs, 1 g dietary fiber, no sugar, and 1 g protein. Oyster: Serving size 1 large. Each serving contains 52 calories, 0.65 g fat, no

	cholesterol, 27 mg sodium, 622 mg potassium, 9.52 g carbs, 3.6 g dietary fiber, 1.64 g sugars, 4.94 g protein.
	Button: Serving size ½ cup. Each serving contains 30 calories, 0.4 g fat, 0 mg cholesterol, 3 g carbs, 2 g dietary fiber, no sugar and 3 g protein.
Okra	Serving size, 1 cup. Each serving contains 31 calories, no cholesterol, 8 mg sodium, 303 mg potassium, 7 g carbs, 3.2 g dietary fiber, 1.2 g sugars, 2 g protein.
Onions	Serving size: 1 tbsp chopped. Each serving contains 4 calories, 0.01 g of total fat, no cholesterol, no sodium, 14 mg potassium, 1.01 g carbs, 0.1 g dietary fiber, 0.43 g sugars, 0.09 g protein.
Parsley	Serving size: 1 tbsp. Each serving contains 1 calorie, 0.03 g total fat, 0 mg cholesterol, 2 mg sodium, 21 mg potassium, 0.24 g carbs, 0.01 g dietary fiber, 0.03 g sugar, 0.11 g protein.
Radicchio	Serving size: 1 cup of shredded. Each serving contains 9 calories, 0.1 g fat, no cholesterol, 9 mg sodium, 121 mg potassium, 1.79 g carbs, 0.4 g dietary fiber, 0.24 g sugars, and 0.57 g protein.
Radishes	Serving size: 1 cup slices. Each serving contains 19 calories, 0.12 g total fat, 0 mg cholesterol, 45 mg sodium, 270 mg potassium, 3.94 g carbs, 1.8 g dietary fiber, 2.46 g sugars, 0.8 g protein.
Rutabaga	
Scallions	Serving size, 1 tbsp chopped. Each serving contains 2 calories. 0.01 g fat, no cholesterol, 1 mg sodium, 17 mg potassium, 0.44 g carbs,

	0.2 g dietary fiber, 0.14 g sugars, 0.11 g protein.
Seaweed (dulse, nori, hikiki, kombu)	Serving size: 1 cup. Each serving contains 30 calories, 0.21 g fat, no cholesterol, 71 mg sodium, 147 mg potassium, 6.74 g carbs, 0.6 g dietary fiber, 0.4 g sugars, 1.9 g protein.
Snow Peas	Serving size: 1 cup of whole pods. Each serving contains 26 calories, 0.13 g fat, no cholesterol, 3 mg sodium, 126 mg potassium, 4.7 g carbs, 1.6 g dietary fiber, 2.5 g sugars, 1.76 g protein.
Spinach	Serving size: 1 cup. Each serving contains 7 calories, 0.12 g fat, no cholesterol, 24 mg sodium, 167 mg potassium, 1.09 g carbs, 0.7 g dietary fiber, 0.87 g protein.
Sprouts (all varieties)	Serving size 1 cup. Each serving contains 16 calories, 0.27 g fat, no cholesterol, 3 mg sodium, 60 mg potassium, 2,6 g carbs, 1.2 g dietary fiber, 1.03 g sugars, 2.01 g protein.
String beans	Serving size: 1 cup. Each serving contains 34 calories, 0.13 g fat, no cholesterol, 7 mg sodium, 230 mg potassium, 7.84 g carbs, 3.7 g dietary fiber, 1.54 g sugars, 2 g protein.
Turnip	Serving size: 1 cup. Each serving contains 36 calories, 0.13 g total fat, no cholesterol, 87 mg sodium, 248 mg potassium, 8.36 g carbs, 2.3 g dietary fiber, 4.94 g sugars, 1.16 g protein.
Water Chestnuts	Serving size: ½ cup. Each serving contains 60 calories, 0.06 g fat, no cholesterol, 9 mg sodium, 362 mg potassium, 14.84 g carbs, 1.9 g dietary fiber, 2.98 g sugars, 0.87 g protein.

Watercress	Serving size: 1 cup chopped. Each serving contains 0.03 g fat, no cholesterol, 14 mg sodium, 112 mg potassium, 0.44 g carbs, 0.3 g dietary fiber, 0.78 g protein.
Zucchini	Serving size, 1 cup chopped. Each serving contains 20 calories, 0.22 g total fat, no cholesterol, 12 mg sodium, 325 mg potassium, 4.15 g carbs, 1.4 g dietary fiber, 2.15 g sugars, 1.5 g protein.

High Fiber Starches	
Tortillas	The nutritional value of these items will vary greatly depending on the manufacturer. Ensure that the ones you choose are high in fiber low in carbs.
Low Carb, high fiber crackers	

Legumes (limited quantities)	
Black Soybeans	The nutritional value of these products varies greatly due to region and methods of manufacturing. Ensure that you choose low carb varieties when possible.
Hummus (as condiment only)	

Coffee Substitutes	
Roma	The nutritional value of these items depends greatly on the manufacturer and how they process their products.
Green Tea	

Herbal Tea	
Condiments, spices, Seasonings	
Basil	The nutritional value of condiments and seasonings will range widely depending on the manufacturer, or where the product is grown. Please refer to the packaging for details about any specific seasoning, seasoning blend or condiment.
Brag's Liquid Aminos	
Cardamom	
Black pepper	It is important to choose products that are low calorie, low carb, and contain high amounts of protein if possible.
Cayenne Pepper	
Capers	
Cajun Blended Seasonings	
Cinnamon	
Crushed red pepper flakes	
Cumin	
Curry powder	
Dill Weed	

Fennel	
Garlic	
Indian blended seasonings	
Lemon	
Lime	
Mexican blended seasonings	
Miso salt	
Mustard	
Nutmeg	
Onion	
Oregano	
Paprika	
Rosemary	
Tamari	
Tarragon	
Thyme	
Vanilla	
Vinegar (balsamic, redwine,	

umeboshi, and rice	
Worchester shire Sauce	

Foods to Be Eaten Only in Moderation and to be avoided for the first 3 weeks (Table 2)

Fats	
Coffee cream	Serving size: 1 tbsp. Each serving contains 20 calories, 1.72 g of fat, 6 mg cholesterol, 6 mg sodium, 20 mg potassium, 0.64 g carbohydrates, no dietary fiber, 0.02 g sugars, and 0.44 g protein.
Canola Oil	Serving size: 1 tsp. Each serving contains 120 calories, 14 g fat, and all other values are 0.
Coconut Oil	Serving size, 1 tbsp. Each serving size contains 117 calories, 13.6 g fat and all other values are 0.
Ghee (clarified butter)	Serving size: 1 tsp. Each serving contains 45 calories, 5 grams fat, 8 mg cholesterol and all other values are 0.
High Oleic Safflower Oil	Serving size 1 tbsp. Each serving contains 120 calories, 13.6 g fat. All other values are 0.
Beef	**Only One Serving Per week. All fat should be trimmed from meat.**
Beef Tenderloin	Serving size, 1 ounce. Each serving contains 43 calories, 1.85 g fat, 19 mg cholesterol, 16 mg sodium, 98 mg potassium, no carbs, no dietary fiber and 6.27 g protein.
Cubed Steak	Serving size: 4 ounces. Each serving contains, 240 calories, 16 g fat, 70 mg cholesterol, 60 mg sodium, no carbs, no dietary fiber, no sugars, 23 g protein.

Filet Mignon	Serving size: 6 ounces. Each serving contains 250 calories, 11 g fat, 115 mg cholesterol, 370 mg sodium, no carbs, no dietary fiber, no sugars, 35 g protein.
Flank Steak	Serving size: 1 ounce. Each serving size contains 53 calories, 1.88 g fat, 19 mg cholesterol, 107 mg sodium, 96 mg potassium, 107 mg sodium, 96 mg potassium, no carbs, no dietary fiber, no sugars, and 8.7 g protein.
Ground Round, Extra Lean	Serving size, 1 patty. Each serving contains 180 calories, 11.7 g fat, 61 mg cholesterol, no carbs, no dietary fiber, no sugar, and 17.35 g protein.
Round Steak Roast beef (top round or rump)	Serving size: 4 ounces. Each serving contains 188 calories, 8.99 g fat, 45 mg cholesterol, 68 mg sodium, 396 mg potassium, no carbs, no dietary fiber, no sugars, 25.02 g protein.
Sirloin Steak	Serving size 5 ounces. Contains 285 calories, 18.02 g fat, 67 mg cholesterol, 74 mg sodium, 447 mg potassium, no carbs, no dietary fiber, no sugars, and 28.78 g protein.
Lamb	**Only one serving per week**
Chop	Serving size: 1 medium 6 ounce. Each serving contains 342 calories, 26.56 g fat, 104 mg cholesterol, 425 mg sodium, 278 mg potassium, no carbs, no dietary fiber, no sugars, 24.01 g protein.
Leg	Serving size, 1 ounce. Each serving contains, 38 calories, 1.44 g fat, 19 mg

	cholesterol, 18 mg sodium, 81 mg potassium, no carbs, no dietary fiber, no sugars, and 5.83 g protein.
Roast	Serving size: 1 thin slice. Each serving contains 37 calories, 2.54 g total fat, 13 mg cholesterol, 32 mg sodium, 39 mg potassium, no carbs, no dietary fiber, no sugars, and 3.35 g protein.

Pork	
Lean, boiled ham	Serving size: one thin slice. Each serving contains 57 calories, 3.8 g of fat, 20 mg of cholesterol, 47 mg of sodium, 74 mg of potassium, no carbs, no dietary fiber, no sugars, and 5.61 g of protein.
Loin Chop	Serving size, 4 ounces. Each serving contains 163 calories, 6.68 mg of cholesterol, 202 mg sodium, 515 mg potassium, no carbs, no dietary fiber, and no sugars, 24.21 g protein.
Pork Tenderloin	Serving size, 4 ounces. Each serving contains 154 calories, 6.13 grams of fat, 75 mg of cholesterol, 56 mg of sodium, 407 mg potassium, no carbs, no dietary fiber, no sugars, and 23.29 g of protein.

Dairy	
Hard Cheese	**Choose light varieties.** (only one slice per day)
Cheddar	Serving size: 1 slice or 1 ounce. Each serving contains 113 calories, 9.28 g fat, 29 mg cholesterol, 174 mg sodium, 27 mg potassium, 0.36 g

	carbs, no dietary fiber, 0.15 g sugars, 6.97 g protein.
Colby	Serving size: 1 slice or 1 ounce. Each serving contains 110 calories, 8.99 g fat, 27 mg cholesterol, 169 mg sodium, 36 mg potassium, 0.72 carbs, no dietary fiber, 0.15 sugars, 6.64 g protein.
Havarti	Serving size, 1 slice or 1 ounce. Each serving contains 105 calories, 8.41 g fat, 27 mg cholesterol, 159 mg sodium, 39 mg potassium, 0.79 g carbs, no dietary fiber, 0.14 g sugars, and 6.49 g protein.
Monterey Jack	Serving size: 1 slice or 1 ounce. Each serving contains 106 calories, 8.85 g fat, 25 mg cholesterol, 152 mg sodium, 23 mg potassium, 0.19 g carbs, no dietary fiber, 0.14 g sugars, 6.94 g protein.
Provolone	Serving size, 1 slice or 1 ounce. Each serving contains 98 calories, 7.45 g total fat, 19 mg cholesterol, 245 mg sodium, 39 mg potassium, 0.6 g carbs, no dietary fiber, 0.16 g sugars, 7.16 g protein.
Swiss	Serving size: 1 slice or 1 ounce. Each serving contains 106 calories, 7.78 g total fat, 26 mg cholesterol, 54 mg sodium, 22 mg potassium, 1.51 g carbs, 0.37 g sugars, 7.54 g protein.
Soft Cheese	
Non-fat plain yogurt	Add one tbsp of flaxseed to increase protein (do not eat more than 2 ½ servings of 1 cup each per week)

	Serving size: 1 cup. Each serving contains 110 calories, no fat, 10 mg cholesterol, 150 mg sodium, 52 mg potassium, 17 g carbs, no dietary fiber, 16 g sugars, 16 g sugars, 11 g protein.
One percent cottage cheese	Serving size ½ cup. Each serving contains 90 calories, 2 g total fat, 5 mg cholesterol, 380 mg sodium, 4 g carbs, 4 g sugar, 15 g protein.
Part Skim Milk Ricotta Cheese	Serving size ¼ cup. Each serving contains 80 calories, 4.5 g fat, 30 mg cholesterol, 60 mg sodium, 100 mg potassium, 4 g carbs, 1 g sugar, 5 g protein.
Carbohydrates	**Do not eat more than ½ cup each day. Avoid these vegetables for the first three weeks of your diet.**
Carrots	Serving size: 1 cup. Each serving contains 52 calories, 0.31 g fat, no cholesterol, 88 mg sodium, 410 mg potassium, 12.26 mg carbs, 3.6 g dietary fiber, 5.81 g sugars, and 1.19 g protein.
Parsnips	Serving size: 1 cup. Each serving contains 100 calories, 0.4 g fat, no cholesterol, 13 mg sodium, 499 mg potassium, 23.92 g carbs, 6.5 g dietary fiber, 6.38 g sugars, 1.6 g protein.
Peas	Serving size: 1 cup. Each serving contains 117 calories, 0.58 g fat, no cholesterol, 7 mg sodium, 354 mg potassium, 20.97 g carbs, 7.4 g dietary fiber, 8.22 g sugars, 7.86 g protein.

Fruit	You should not eat more than 1 serving per day. Do not eat canned fruit. You should only eat fresh or frozen.
Apples	Serving size: 1 medium apple. Each serving contains 95 calories, 0.3 g fat, 0 mg cholesterol, 2 mg sodium, 195 mg potassium, 25 g carbs, 4.4 g dietary fiber, 19 g sugar, 0.5 g protein.
Apricots	Serving size: 2 cup sliced. Each serving contains 79 calories, 0.6 g fat, 0 cholesterol, 2 mg sodium, 427 mg potassium, 18 g carbs, 3.3 g dietary fiber, 15 g sugar, and 2.3 g protein.
Blueberries	Serving size: 1 cup. Each serving contains 85 calories, 0.5 g fat, no cholesterol, 1 mg sodium, 114 mg potassium, 21 g carbs, 3.6 g dietary fiber, 15 g sugar, 1.1 g protein.
Cherries	Serving size: 1 cup without pits. Each serving contains 77 calories, 0.5 g fat, o cholesterol, 5 mg sodium, 268 mg potassium, 19 g carbs, 2.5 g dietary fiber, 13 g sugar, 1.6 g protein.
Grapes	Serving size: 1 cup. Each serving contains 62 calories, 0.3 g fat, no cholesterol, 2 mg sodium, 176 mg potassium, 16 g carbs, 0.8 g dietary fiber, 15 g sugar, 0.6 g protein.
Kiwi	Serving size: 1 fruit. Each serving contains 42 calories, 0.4 g fat, no cholesterol, 2 mg sodium, 215 mg potassium, 10 g carbs, 2.1 g dietary fiber, 6 g sugar, 0.8 g protein.
Nectarines	Serving size: 1 medium. Each serving contains 59 calories, 0.4 g fat, no

	cholesterol, no sodium, 285 mg potassium, 14 g carbs, 2.2 g dietary fiber, 13 g sugar, and 1.4 g protein.
Peaches	Serving size: 1 medium. Each serving contains 59 calories, 0.4 g fat, no cholesterol, no sodium, 285 mg potassium, 14 g carbs, 2.2 g dietary fiber, 13 g sugar, and 1.4 g protein.
Pears	Serving size: 1 medium. Each serving contains 102 calories, 0.2 g fat, no cholesterol, 2 mg sodium, 206 mg potassium, 27 carbs, 6 g dietary fiber, 17 g sugar, 0.6 g protein.
Plums	Serving size: 1 fruit. Each serving contains 30 calories, 0.2 g fat, 0 cholesterol, 0 sodium, 104 mg potassium, 8 g carbs, 0.8 g dietary fiber, 7 g sugar, 0.5 g protein.
Raspberries	Serving size: 1 cup. Each serving contains 65 calories, 0.8 g fat, no cholesterol, 1 mg sodium, 185 g potassium, 15 g carbs, 8 g dietary fiber, 5 g sugar, and 1.5 g protein.
Strawberries	Serving size: 1 medium. Each serving contains 4 calories, no fat, no cholesterol, no sodium, 18 mg potassium, 0.9 grams carbs, 0.2 g dietary fiber, 0.6 g sugar, 0.1 g protein.
Tomatoes	Serving size: 1 medium whole. Each serving contains 22 calories, 0.2 g of fat, no cholesterol, 5 mg sodium, 292 mg potassium, 4.8 g carbs, 1.5 g dietary fiber, 3.3 g sugar, 1.1 g protein.
Seeds	Seeds should be raw, unroasted, and unsalted nuts are best.

Pumpkin	
Poppy	
Sesame	
Sesame Tahini	
Sunflower	
Legumes	
Adzuki	
Navy	
Lentil	
Mung	
Low Carb Tomato Sauce	Any brand with 5 or less grams of carbs
Beverages	
1 cup of real coffee	
4 ounces of red wine	A serving of red wine, or 4 ounces of red wine, contains 80 calories. It also contains, 1 mg of sodium, and 1 g of carbohydrates.
Sweeteners (limited quantity)	
Stevia	Serving size is 1 packet. Each packet contains 1 calorie, 1 g of carbs and 1 g of dietary fiber.

Foods To Be Completely Avoided (Table 3)

Dairy	Off-Limits Legumes	Off Limits Fats
Milk	Chickpeas (other than a small amount of hummus)	All commercially processed oils
Frozen custard	Lima beans	Hydrogenated fats
Frozen yogurt	Peanuts	Lard
Fruit-flavored yogurt	Peanut butter	Margarines containing Transfatty acids
Ice cream	Pinto beans	Peanut oil
All Full-Fat Hard Cheeses		Soybean oil
Cheddar	**Vegetables**	Sunflower oil
Colby	Corn and corn products	Squeezable butter
Havarti	White potatoes	Shortening
Monterey Jack	Pumpkin	
Provolone	Yams	**Sugar and Artificial Sweeteners**
Swiss		Brown Sugar
	Bad Condiments	Corn Syrup
Meats	Barbecue sauce	Dextrose
Chicken Roll	Most commercially prepared salad dressing	Fructose

Corned Beef	Ketchup	Honey
Honey Turkey	Mayonnaise	Maple Sugar
Hotdogs (all)		Nutrasweet
Pastrami	**Beverages**	Saccharin
Sandwich Meats	Fruit juice	Sucrose
Sausage (other than turkey or chicken)	Soda	Sugar
Turkey Roll	Sports drinks	Sweet'n low
Roast Beef	Sweetened teas	Tubinado
All Fried Foods	**Starches**	**Snack Foods**
Fried Chicken	Bread	Chips
Fried Fish	Couscous	Breakfast bars
Chicken Nuggets	Crackers	Energy bars
French Fries	Muffins	Cakes
	Packaged pancake mix	Candy
Fruits	Packaged dry cereal	Cookies
Banana	Pasta	Flavored jell-o
Cantaloupe	Rice	Frozen fruit ice

Dried Fruit	Quinoa	Gelato
Grapes	Waffles	Ice cream
Honeydew		Popcorn
Orange		Pretzels
Pineapple		
Watermelon		

Conclusion

Leptin resistance is created when the brain no longer recognizes the chemical hormone leptin in the blood. Leptin is secreted by fat cells. In the leptin-resistant state, the brain has no way of knowing how much fat the body has stored since it can no longer measure the chemical.

Modern medicine cannot reverse this disorder on its own. Even though there are two medications used to help reduce the amount of body fat stored, they cannot make the body more receptive to the chemical itself. The only way to reverse leptin resistance is through diet, exercise, proper sleep, and supplementation.

In order to change your body, you must be willing to change several aspects in your life. You must be willing to change your diet, increase your exercise, monitor the way your body feels, and make adjustments as needed.

The leptin resistance diet is high in omega-3s, dietary fiber, and empty calories. Because of this, you should not follow this diet for a prolonged period of time. The diet should be followed for a maximum of six weeks. If you plan to lose more weight, you should take a two-week break before starting again.

The leptin-resistant diet follows some of the same general principals of a diabetic diet. If you have a confirmed diagnosis of leptin resistance, it is important to be tested for diabetes and other related illnesses, as they are known to coexist.

The recipes in this book are only for starter purposes. There are thousands of recipes to help aid in reversing leptin resistance. You can create your own by following the food chart in this book.

Best of luck!

Christine Weil

Check out the other books in the *Natural Health & Natural Cures Series*

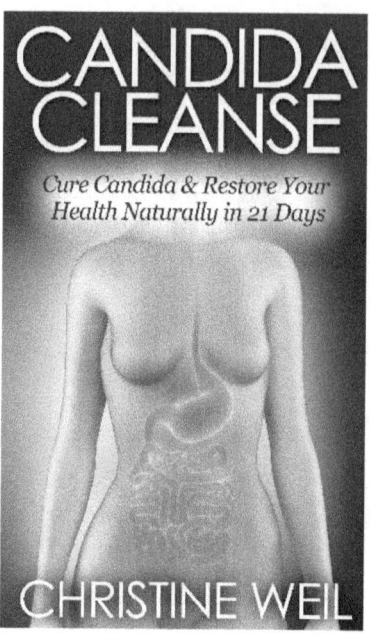

http://www.amazon.com/dp/B00IIRQH9K

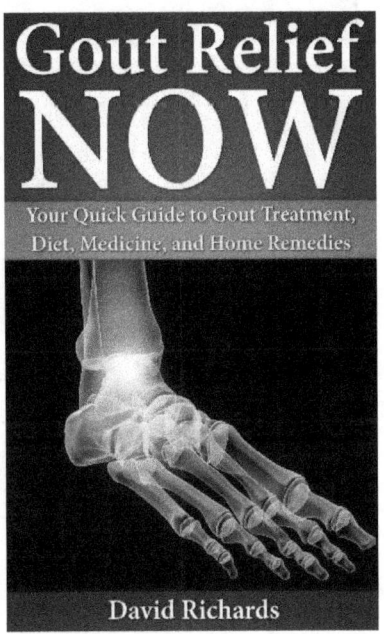

http://www.amazon.com/dp/B00HHGRBBQ

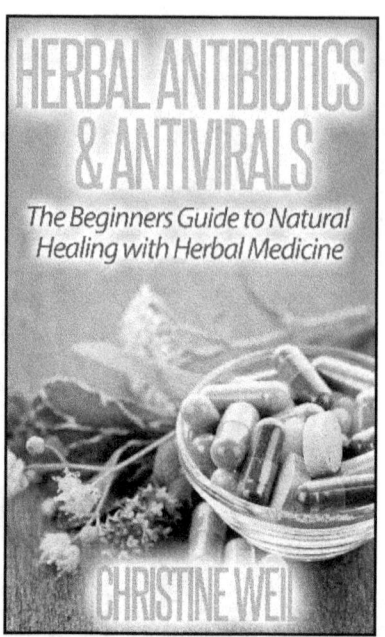

http://www.amazon.com/dp/B00J2F1QDO

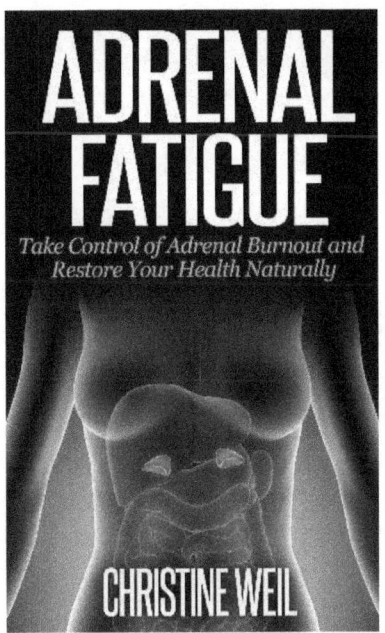

http://www.amazon.com/dp/B00J8SHS6E

www.ingramcontent.com/pod-product-compliance
Lightning Source LLC
Chambersburg PA
CBHW071624170526
45166CB00003B/1180